Living the Fat Burning Lifestyle

Make These Key Changes to Rev Up Your Metabolism and Burn Fat Passively!

Ron Kness

Published by:

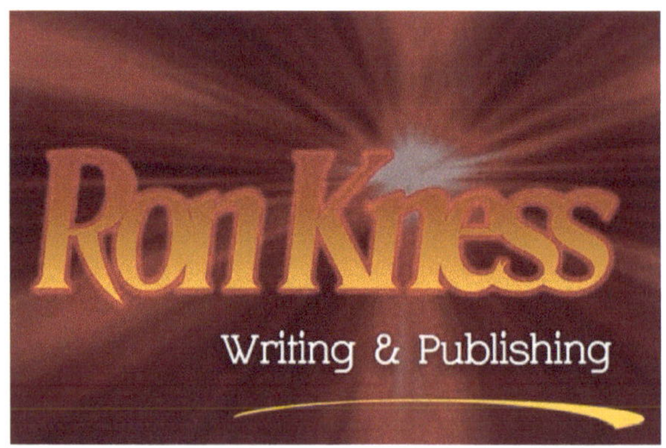

https://ronknesswriting.com

Ron Kness

Queen Creek, AZ

United States of America

ISBN: 9781710900736

Sneak Peek

For anyone trying to lose weight, it can be frustrating to see the scale refuse to budge or to feel weak and tired all the time because of your diet. If you want to rev up your weight loss efforts, though, you should focus on burning more fat, which is excess weigh your body does not need. By getting rid of fat, you will feel better, your clothes will fit more loosely, and you will finally start to see a different number on that scale.

While your body normally wants to burn fat as an energy source, there are ways that you can improve its capacity to do so, turning your body into a fat-burning machine that can help you lose weight. By changing some strategies for improving your ability to burn fat, including ways you can change your exercise routine and diet as well as other parts of your lifestyle, you can boost your ability to get rid of that extra fat.

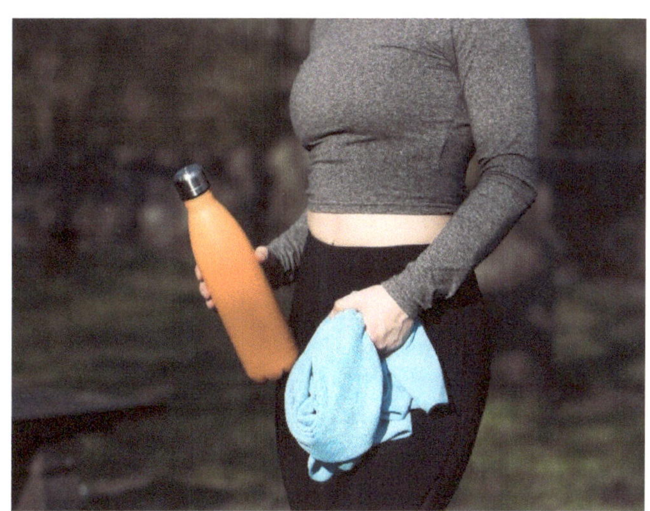

It is vital you understand the role of fat for your health and how your body actually burns the stored fat you are carting around. Knowing how you use the food you eat to fuel your body can help you make better choices about what you put in your mouth as well as how you move your body.

You get the energy your body needs from the fat, carbohydrates, and proteins, which are in the foods you eat. Your body draws from various sources depending on its energy needs and what is available to it. You may think that eating less fat, for example, will cause your body to burn your stored fat instead. In reality, that is not always true.

3

When your body needs quick energy, such as while you are doing intense exercise or while you are actively working, it will go first to carbohydrates as its source of fuel. Carbs are easy to break down, provide a quick burst of fuel, and can give you energy at consistent rates.

Protein is only used for energy when you are using your muscles in powerful ways, as the amino acids that make up these foods are used to repair muscle damages. Fat is burned when your body needs longer, slower stores of energy. This is because fat takes longer to process, and it consumes more energy in the process of creating energy.

Metabolism Basics

You have probably heard about metabolism and that it is essential for losing weight and burning fat. Your metabolism is not just one thing; it is a complex process that involves many parts of the body that govern the chemical processes and hormones that keep you alive and ensure you have enough energy to perform necessary tasks. There are many bodily functions that contribute to your metabolism.

Your metabolism exists to keep you alive. It is in charge of converting the food you eat into the energy you can use right now as well as storing excesses into reserves that you can use later. The energy from your diet is used to allow you to pump blood throughout your body, to move and think, to breathe, and to do all the things necessary to keep you alive and healthy.

Your metabolism, as most people refer to it, is actually your resting metabolic rate, which is how well you burn calories to support your basic bodily needs while at rest.

This rate does not consider other activities, such as exercise, performing daily tasks, digesting your food, or anything else. It is basically the energy you need to breathe, pump blood, and for your cells to perform their functions.

This resting rate accounts for about 70 percent of your overall caloric needs. When you alter this rate, you increase your ability to lose weight, burn excess fat, and improve your overall health.

Because a higher total weight means more calories needed to maintain normal function, so the heavier you are, the higher your resting metabolic rate is. That is why, when you lose weight, your metabolic rate decreases because you need fewer calories to live.

Now that we have explored the basics of how you gain and lose weight, we will dive right into our best strategies for boosting fat loss and improving your health!

Disclaimer

This publication is for informational purposes only and is not intended as medical advice. Medical advice should always be obtained from a qualified medical professional for any health conditions or symptoms associated with them.

Every possible effort has been made in preparing and researching this material. We make no warranties with respect to the accuracy, applicability of its contents or any omissions.

See your healthcare professional before starting any diet, health or exercise program!

Contents

Introduction

Hello and welcome to our short, beginners guide on how to finally lose the excess weight and keep it off forever by making little key changes in your lifestyle.

Firstly, I've got some great news for you: most diets work – at least in the short-term. But very few work over the long-term. To lose weight and keep it off for good, you need to switch to a healthy eating lifestyle – one you can live on for the rest of your life.

I know that sounds crazy because you are reading this book for a good reason. You're reading this book because you've gone on several diets in the past and you didn't get the results that you were looking for.

Well, the truth is, if we're completely honest about it, most diets do work. Seriously. Diets do produce the weight loss that they claim, plus or minus a few pounds here and there.

What's missing from the picture is the fact that diets are really products of the market. They're not much different from stuff that you can buy in any grocery store.

These diets books and weight loss programs are commercial products, and guess what? Just like any commercial product, they won't sell if, at some level or another, they don't work. Let's just put it that way.

Diets that become popular, like the Paleo diet, the **Ketogenic diet**, the Atkins diet, and others that are out there, became popular precisely because they work. That's the good news. Here's the bad news: diets do work but they work initially.

What do I mean by that? When you get on a diet, you lose weight for a few weeks, and then all of a sudden, the weight loss starts to slow down. It then stops. And before you're fully aware of it, all that weight comes back.

This is the bad news that few people rarely see publicized in the media. And for good reason. There's no money in it.

The sad reality is that most dieters gain their weight back. It doesn't matter how much weight they lost initially. It doesn't matter how rapidly they lost weight. It's going to come back. Worse yet, they weigh even more after they end their diet.

Imagine that. You put in all this time to lose weight, you did the right things, and then for all your time and trouble, you weigh more than when you began. It's as if all that initial weight that you lost came rushing back to your midsection, and they brought their friends with them. Pretty depressing, right?

Well, it is quite demotivating, and that's why a lot of people simply get discouraged. They try one diet after another, only to experience the same sad results. They've seen this movie over and over again. It is a hamster wheel that they just can't get off of!

The #1 Challenge with Diets

Let me be clear, the number one challenge with diets is not whether you're going to experience weight loss or not. The truth is, weight loss will happen. Any diet worth its salt is going to deliver weight loss.

The challenge with most diets also doesn't have anything to do with timelines. Given enough time, you will lose weight.

Interestingly enough, the challenge doesn't involve any kind of difficulty because most diets out there are actually pretty straightforward when it comes to their requirements. As long as you follow them step by step, you will get the results that you are looking for; again, give or take a few pounds here and there.

Granted, some diets are easier to follow than others, but generally speaking, when it comes to difficulty, most weight loss programs are not all that hard. The challenge doesn't involve the difficulty of losing weight.

Where the Challenge Lies

So, what is the number one challenge with diets? Let me pull the cat out of the bag: it's all about sustainability.

Until and unless scientists are somehow, some way, able to pack discipline, self-control and willpower in a capsule form, the number one challenge with diets, and any other kind of weight loss program for that matter, will be sustainability.

It doesn't really matter how much weight you lose at first. If you know full well that you're going to regain that weight, then you're just wasting your time.

It's hard for people to be consistent with their diet. They think they're making all this progress. They look in the mirror and they see a much better-looking person, and then all of a sudden, after a few weeks, they can't help themselves and they slowly but surely get back to their old weight.

Does this sound depressing? Do you feel discouraged or demotivated? I've got some good news for you. This book will help you finally break that cycle.

Make no mistake, a lot of people are going through the same thing you are. There is a multibillion-dollar diet industry that depends on people like you failing. That's why the global weight loss industry is so lucrative.

People like yourself go from one diet to another. They buy book after book, and sign up for one weight loss program after another. In fact, the whole gym membership industry is built on this expectation of failure.

If you're sick and tired of failing, you are reading the right book. If you follow the tips that I will share with you in this book, you will finally be able to break this multibillion-dollar weight loss scam cycle once and for all.

Chapter 1 – Be Clear On How Weight Loss Actually Works

One of the biggest obstacles to sustainable weight loss is the fact that a lot of people have this magical thinking about diets. They think that it's all about the diet itself, how it helps you skip certain foods, or how it magically boosts the amount of fat you burn in any given day.

No wonder people fail with their diets because they don't have a clear picture of how fat is actually burned by the human body.

If you don't have that basic working understanding, then it's very easy for you to engage in lifestyle choices that will eventually lead you to undermine whatever progress you make.

Let me simplify things to its most basic terms in this chapter. This way, you can have a good working understanding of how weight loss actually works so you can make better informed decisions as far as your lifestyle goes.

Weight Loss is All About Calories In and Calories Out

While there are metabolic dynamics that complicate how quickly you lose weight, weight loss is basically all about calorie accounting at the end of the day.

It's actually quite basic. To lose weight, the number of calories you ingest in any given day must be less than the calories you burn for that day.

On the flipside, if you want to gain weight, you have to burn fewer calories than the amount of calories you eat.

For people trying to lose weight, I've got some great news. Your body is actually a calorie-burning machine. If you don't believe me, think of the things that you normally do "automatically."

All of us have to breathe, digest our food, go to the bathroom, pump blood through our system, blink, and other seemingly "automatic actions." Do you think these things happen magically without any kind of energy source? Absolutely not. Every breath you take as you read this book burns calories.

The truth is, every single moment you're alive, you are burning calories. For your body to maintain a certain temperature, you have to burn calories. That's the good news.

The bad news is that the number of calories you eat every single day must be below the amount of calories you burn. If you eat more calories than your body burns, your body stores the excess energy in the form of fat.

You're not a plant, so your body doesn't store energy in the form of starch. The white sticky stuff that you get from rice, that's stored energy. The same goes with the sugary mass you get from corn or potatoes.

Plants store energy in the form of starch. Animals, such as human beings, store excess energy in the form of fat.

Most Stored Fat Starts Out as Blood Sugar

To get a clear understanding of how weight loss works, you have to first be clear on how your body uses energy as well as what kind of forms of energy it usually uses.

Generally speaking, your body burns sugar for energy. This pretty much applies to most people. There are certain people that burn fat for energy, and I will get to that. But generally speaking, when you talk to the average American, their body uses the sugar in their bloodstream for energy.

Are you with me so far? Good.

Now, when your body can't burn the sugar in your bloodstream because there is simply too much sugar, it will try to do two things. First, your body will try to pass that extra sugar as waste. If that doesn't happen, the excess is converted by your liver into fat, which is then stored in your fat cells.

Please understand that a human body has a certain fixed number of fat cells. But just because you have all those fat cells, it doesn't necessarily mean you're fat. Your body has to fill those cells with fat molecules for you to look fat and to weigh more.

Weight Loss is All About Triggering a Net Negative Calorie State

As I've mentioned earlier, for you to lose weight, your body has to burn more calories than the calories that it's taking in. In other words, if your body doesn't have enough calories to cover its energy requirements, you start to lose weight.

How does this happen? Well, first of all, your body starts to unlock the water in your system. You lose water, and this translates into heavy initial weight loss.

If you've ever gone on the Keto, Paleo, or Atkins diet, a lot of the initial weight loss that you enjoy at first is actually water leaving your system.

When you switch mostly to fat-based diet or protein-based diet, this means there's less carbohydrates in your system. Carbohydrates absorb quite a bit of water. So, when you switch to a protein or fat-based diet, a lot of the carbohydrates in your bloodstream is flushed out and a lot of water goes with it.

However, if you're looking for more sustainable weight loss, and I would dare say "real" weight loss, you have to start burning fat for energy. This is the long-term solution for weight loss. We'll get to how to trigger this process in a later chapter in this book.

At this point, I just want you to be clear on how weight loss actually works so you can make an informed decision as to how to alter your lifestyle in a painless way so you can turn your body into a fat-burning machine.

Excited yet? Good. Meet me at Chapter 2.

Chapter 2 -Why Most Diets Fail

Most weight loss programs fail because of their lack of sustainability.

They don't fail because they're ineffective. They don't fail because they're badly designed. They don't fail because they have their biochemistry wrong. Let's get that out of the way.

It has nothing to do with their overall effectiveness. It's all about sustainability. And where is sustainability centered? Sadly, it's centered on you.

It's all about your willpower. Are you willing to stick with something for the long term? Are you willing to commit to certain lifestyle changes required by the diet that you chose so you can keep the weight off? This is where people fall short.

The bottom line is, most people can't just sustain a diet for a long-term period. They may jump in with both feet because they're pumped up at first, especially if they enjoy a tremendous amount of weight loss, but sooner or later, they hit a plateau.

Unless you're careful, sooner or later, the weight comes back. If you are particularly unlucky, which most of us tend to be, you end up weighing more.

Most Diets are Not Sustainable Because They are Alien to Us

I've got some bad news. I don't care how excited you are about the diet that you're thinking of getting on. I don't care about how pumped up many people are around you regarding that diet. The truth is, most diets are alien to us.

They push us to eat one type of food over another. They require such drastic portion control. They even insist that you cut out certain classes of food entirely from your diet.

Don't get me wrong, I'm not saying that you are unable to do this at first. Most people are so desperate for a solution that they are able to do it. The question is, you have to ask yourself, "What happens next?"

Unfortunately, the typical diet is like some sort of imposition. It's just not part of who you are. You've grown accustomed to certain tastes; you are very familiar with a certain eating lifestyle, so what happens is you're pushed to eat less of the food you like.

This is the food that helps you define your identity. This is the kind of food that you simply grew up with or it's just simply part of you. And, to make matters worse, the typical diet usually shifts you to a class of food that you normally don't eat.

I'm not just talking about vegan or vegetarian diets. There are other diet modifications like the **Paleo diet** that people simply are not all that familiar with.

Now, if you ask them, they make a big deal out of the fact that they're eating more meat so they're excited. But deep down inside, they're unfamiliar. They're not really accustomed to it.

So eventually, this disconnect between what you're used to and the new diet that you're on will come to the surface as food cravings, and guess what? You're going to lose out – every time. You're simply not used to the change.

And that my friend is the essence of why diets fail is because most of them don't allow certain types of food that your body is uses to having. It will put up with not having that food for a while, but eventually it will demand it and you will give in.

The Bottom Line: Most Diets Fail Because Your Body and Mind Fight Back

This is not just a simple matter of being uncomfortable or not getting used to something. Eventually, this disconnect that I'm talking about pits your body and mind against your willpower.

The sad reality is that if you leave your body and mind unchanged and unmodified, they will push back. It may not happen tomorrow or the day after, but it's eventually going to reach a boiling point.

There is such a thing as Regression to the Mean. We just go back to what we're accustomed to. We just go back to the **lifestyle** that we've always known.

What makes this really tragic and somewhat depressing is that it involves a lot of self-sabotage. You know that you should be eating a certain type of food, but you trick yourself into believing that, "Hey, if I can cheat one day, that'll be okay" or "I owe it to myself anyway. I'm just being kind to myself." You rattle off a million and one excuses why you should get off the program.

Well, let me tell you, that one cheat day turns into a cheat week. That cheat week turns into a cheat month. And before you know it, you're completely off the program.

This self-sabotage is real and it's insidious precisely because it happens below the surface. You don't look at yourself in the mirror and say, "Well, I don't really like myself. I don't really like the program that I'm on. I'm going to sabotage myself."

It's not that obvious. But sooner or later, you find excuses to get off this new programming or new lifestyle and you end up where you began.

The worst part? You become fatter when you get there.

Chapter 3 – Burn Fat By Changing Your Mindset

Considering how dangerous and seemingly self-defeating the whole weight loss program may be because of the level of intrusion most diets pose, what can you do to lose fat sustainably?

The first place to look to when you've decided to finally get serious about losing weight permanently is your **mindset**.

Again, like with most weight loss programs and diet books, mindset is not even talked about. In fact, when you read a typical diet book, it doesn't even talk about having the right expectations, assumptions, and mindset coming into the diet process. It makes the assumption that since you're reading this diet book, you already have the right mindset.

Well, let's take a step back and understand why most people fail with their diets. The sad reality is that when people go on a diet, they adopt a diet mindset. What is this mindset? What truths does it yield when we break it apart?

Well, first of all, they assume that they're about to do something that is ultimately temporary. When you ask a person that is about to go on a diet, whether it's the Paleo diet, the Atkins diet, the South Beach diet, they would tell you that they're excited about the diet. But the subtext of what they're doing, as far as their attitudes go, is that "This is temporary. This is not really me. This is just a stage in my life or a solution to a problem that I have."

The next assumption, which is closely related to the first one, is that "This is alien to me."

In other words, it's not much different from the alien that tore through the chest of that hapless astronaut in the classic sci-fi movie "Alien." Most of us are not born with an alien in our chest poking a hole through our heart.

Believe it or not, on a subconscious level, most people think that the diet they're on is strange to them. It is not natural to them. It is not something that they would normally choose. I hope you can see the picture here.

When you go on a diet, your mindset is looking at what you're doing as something that's temporary, so it's not really part of a long-term personal evolution. It's looking at the changes that you're going to go through as something that's fundamentally strange. It's not part of you.

You look at it as something that doesn't normally flow from how you look at things or how you normally eat. So, what happens? The first few weeks, your body accommodates these changes because hey, you're pumped up.

Maybe you looked in the mirror and you just felt that you had to lose weight because something has to be done. You feel desperate. So. you lose a lot of weight in the beginning, but eventually, there will be a pushback.

That accommodation leads to a pushback because you're doing something that, deep down inside, you feel that you shouldn't normally do. Why? It's not part of you. You're doing something strange. You're doing something weird.

Think of Your Fat-Burning Diet as Part of Your Routine

Thankfully, there is an alternative to the typical diet mindset. When you decide to finally get off the weight loss treadmill, you can choose to start looking at these lifestyle changes and modified decisions as part of your routine.

In other words, you're looking at food selection as part of who you are. This is not something that's imposed on you, this is not something that comes outside of you, but is really just an extension of who you already are. Do you see the difference?

This is why one of the first steps that you need to take to burn fat sustainably is to displace, not replace. In other words, instead of just waking up one day and saying, "Okay, I'm not going to drink any more soda" or "I'm not going to do this" or "I'm not going to eat that," you simply add to your plate.

You're pumped up about a new weight loss system so you take the foods in that system and you add it to your routine. You don't cut anything out. This leads to displacement.

How? Well, you think of the small changes to your diet as enhancing or adding or supplementing your existing habits.

There's no threat in this. Your body and mind complex don't see this as an imposition or some sort of ordeal. It doesn't feel like you're punishing yourself or you're somehow, some way, being left behind. Instead, you're just adding to what you're already doing.

Compare this with the typical diet where you cut out certain foods almost overnight. You feel like you're challenging yourself, eroding what's already there, and this leads to a sense of threat. Believe me, your psychology picks up on this. It doesn't scream it out at you, but it is obvious.

The assumption then, when you choose to displace rather than replace, is that these changes are permanent: I'm simply adding on or enhancing or rediscovering certain things that I already like. This then leads to a more profound assumption, which is "These changes are part of who I am."

I hope you can see the 180-degree difference between this approach with the typical diet mindset.

Prepare to Make Changes and Adapt

A lot of weight loss success really depends on our attitude. When you ask the typical person on a diet if they were to give you an honest answer what motivated them to get on that weight loss program, they would tell you that they were operating at some level of desperation.

Again, I'm talking about people who are completely honest. If you were to read between the lines and peel off a lot of the niceties, this is the bottom line.

Basically, their mindset when they got on that diet is, "I better lose weight or I quit." There's a sense of do or die in their mindset because they look at the diet essentially as a tool to an objective.

Remember, they're thinking that the diet is temporary. That it's just a means to an end.

If you want to be successful with your fat-burning lifestyle change, you have to lose that mindset. This is not a question of do or die, or hit it or quit it. Instead, this is a question of rediscovering who you are or enhancing what you already have.

If you're able to make this mental pivot, then you would be able to prepare to slip up. Remember, anything in life that is worth having is going to be a challenge.

When you went to college, I'm sure there were a few exams that you went through that were not very pretty. You had to deal with those challenges. But if you have a degree, it means you stuck with it.

The same applies to a weight loss lifestyle. If you want to burn fat sustainably, be prepared to slip up.

The problem is, a lot of people on a diet think that it's the diet itself that guarantees success. That if they do A and not B, then they will enjoy C. Not quite.

The truth is, sustainable weight loss is a journey. Not just a journey in terms of you getting acclimated to a new way of eating and allowing your taste buds to evolve, it also involves changing your mindset and perspective. And one of the most important points of adaptation is the willingness to slip up.

Now, keep in mind that preparing to slip up is very different from expecting or wanting to slip up. I'm not saying that you should want to slip up or want to fail. I'm not advocating self-sabotage here. Instead, I am saying that you should have an expectation that you're doing something profound. You're doing something new.

It is difficult, so give yourself a break and understand that you will slip up. But the difference is, when that slip up does happen, you're prepared for it.

How do you prepare? Well, you resolve to get back up.

Let me tell you, the first time you get knocked off track, it's really difficult to get back with the program. But the good news is, the more you get knocked off and get back up, the shorter and shorter that time gap between setback and recovery will be.

This really all boils down to a question of trust. You really don't trust yourself all that much when you get faced with a challenge and you choose to remain down.

Why? You don't trust yourself enough to learn from the experience to do a better job next time, so you stay down. Let me tell you, the only way to lose is if you choose to remain down.

So, understand that this change that you're going through so your body can burn fat like a machine, is a test of your ability to adapt and scale up.

Now, you may be thinking to yourself, "I haven't really adapted." Well, if that's your thinking, I want you to just remember the times you learned certain things in your life.

Think back to when you were learning to ride a bike or swim. The first time you tried, it was not a pretty sight. Maybe you skinned your knee, maybe you almost drowned, but you kept at it. Before you knew it, you adapted. And then you scaled up.

If you're like most people, when you first start to learn how to ride a bike, you probably were swerving all over the place. But as you get used to it and adapted fully, you started pedaling in a straight line.

Let me ask you a question. If you were able to adapt in those situations, what's stopping you from adapting to a fat-burning lifestyle today?

There is really not much difference. In fact, what you're trying to do now is a little bit easier because adapting to bike riding is painful. I know. I have the scars to prove it.

What Mental State Should You Be Aiming For?

Now that we know the negative impact of mindset on weight loss, particularly when it comes to diets, what is the alternative? Well, the mental state that you should be aiming for should be one of relaxation.

Chill out. It's not that hard. People have done it before you. It's not like you're going to the moon and you're doing something that humanity hasn't done before.

People have lost weight and kept it off, so relax. You're not doing the impossible here.

Next, you have to accept what lies ahead. What lies ahead is not a straight line between Point A and Point B. This is not a slam dunk nor is this a guaranteed journey. Instead, it is a journey of discovery and it is a journey filled with challenges.

By understanding that you are going on a journey, you can present yourself with two choices. Either this is going to be a long series of punishments, ordeals and tortures, or it can be a long series of puzzles, problems to be solved, and opportunities to tap into your ability to solve problems and your ability to get inspired.

If you're able to make this transition, your overall mental state would be one of hopefulness and optimism.

You have to think back to when you learned to ride a bike. It would have been so easy to just look at the difficulty of learning to ride a bike and write it off as leading to future pain, loss, scarring, and torture. Believe me, some people have phobias because they developed that mindset. Sustained weight loss can be like that too … if you let it. But with a positive can-do mindset, you can do this!

But you could be like most people and realize that those gashes on your knee form the price you have to pay for that nice, awesome bike ride at the beach right before the sun sets. It all boils down to your mindset. While losing weight is physical in nature, it is also very much mental – something that many people trying to lose weight don't realize.

I'm telling you, if you're aware of the mental state that you should aim for, it's much easier to be hopeful and optimistic because everything worth having requires some sort of sacrifice. There's always some level of doubt or some price you have to pay before you achieve the reward that you desire.

Personally, I look at any kind of learning experience as some sort of neat grand puzzle. It's challenging and it takes a lot of time.

If you break everything down into one puzzle at a time, it's not only doable, but it's also a lot of fun. If anything, it's a journey as to how creative, inventive, resourceful, and clever you really are.

Chapter 4 - Burn Fat by Eating More of the Foods You Like... Strategically

I know a lot of dieticians will probably get into trouble by saying that people looking to lose weight should eat more.

I know it seems like it's some sort of blasphemy or sacrilege, but the truth is, the number one factor that leads to diet failure is the perception that they're doing something that is completely alien to their lifestyle. They're doing something that's simply off the beaten track.

Part of them even warns them that they shouldn't be doing it at all because they are way beyond their comfort zone. This is where the advice of eating more of the foods you like start to make sense.

First, you have to zero in on your favorite tastes. Identify the foods that you think you like. Test yourself and go without those foods for a few days. Can you confirm that you really like those foods?

Maybe you like the condiment, not the main dish. Maybe you like the side dish or the appetizers instead of the main dish. Whatever it is, do a lot of experiments with yourself until you can identify and confirm that you like certain foods because of a certain taste profile.

At this level, you're just looking for the taste profile that you prefer. Some people have a sweet tooth, other people like oily and salty food, others like spicy food. There's really no right or wrong answer. What's important is that you get an accurate read of what your natural favorite taste ranges are.

Identify Your Favorite Dishes

Now that you have a clearer understanding of what your favorite tastes or range of tastes are, the next step is to track all the dishes that you normally eat in a given month. I know this sounds like some sort of record-keeping nightmare, but believe me, you'll get used to it.

Your food journal doesn't have to be anything fancy. You don't have to cut and paste pictures of dishes and recipes and ingredients. There's no need to do that. Just write down the dishes that you eat every single day. Keep in mind that this includes snacks.

At the end of the month, you would be able identify your favorite dishes. Now that you have zeroed in this, you can correlate them with your preferred tastes.

Also, when you have clearly identified what your favorite dishes are, you would also be able to know what your favorite textures are. This is very important.

A lot of people think that when it comes to food, the only thing that matters is taste. Absolutely wrong. People prefer one dish over the other, not just because it tastes different, but it also has a different aroma or it has a different texture. So, you have to factor in these other elements so you can have a more accurate listing of your favorite dishes.

Identify Your Preferred Portions

After one month of tracking your favorite dishes, the next step is to identify your favorite dishes and pay close attention to your portions. In particular, I want you to ask yourself how much do you have to eat of a particular food item until you feel "full"?

This may seem like a very basic question, but if you pay close attention to it and you really track it, you would realize that there are two things going on here. There is physical satiety where you feel physically full, and then there's mental satiety.

I can't even begin to tell you how many times I felt hungry when I'm physically full. Like I can't stuff any more food in my stomach but I still feel that there's something missing.

The flipside can also be true. You can feel full, but there's almost nothing in your stomach. So, understand the difference and then apply this difference to how you track your eating habits.

Identify Your Hydration Points

After you have identified your preferred portions, the next step is to map out when you normally drink before, during and after a meal. This is a very important piece of information to have because this can help you reduce hunger.

Did you know that a lot of people feel hungry but they're not really hungry? How come? Well, it only takes one glass of water to get rid of that hunger.

I know it sounds crazy, but you'd be surprised as to how much of your hunger goes away when you choose to drink one or two glasses of water. For this to happen, you have to know what your ideal hydration points are.

Make Each Meal a Celebration

I remember when I first started work at a big corporation, a couple of friends of mine would always go to this Italian restaurant a block away from out office building. Not only was it convenient, but it was also one of the few places in town that offered authentic Tuscan cuisine.

As you can well imagine, the meals from that place carried a pretty hefty price tag. It is no wonder that my coworkers were quite shocked when they saw me scarf down one bowl of pasta after another.

Finally, one of my friends, Max, got the nerve to ask, "Dude what are you doing?" I said, "Well, I'm eating. We only have an hour and a half to get back to work so I figured I'd load up quick."

Max then went on to explain to me that this type of Italian food is something that you enjoy. In other words, you savor it. It's a celebration. The flavors are to be relished in one's mouth. The texture is to be experienced as one chews.

I thought Max was just being fanciful, but he was absolutely right. Come to think of it, I was paying a large chunk of my paycheck for premium grade food, but I was treating it like it was a McDonald's meal. I didn't see the disconnect. Now I do.

You should apply the same analysis to your meals. It doesn't really matter how much money you spend on your meal. The meal should be a celebration. Each mealtime should be an opportunity for you to truly enjoy your food.

Eating is not just a simple act of opening that hole in your mouth, plowing some nutrients in it, gulping down, chasing it down with some type of liquid, and then calling it a day. When you eat, a lot of your senses are actually involved.

When you eat, it's obvious that your sense of taste is engaged. But you shouldn't also forget that your food looks a certain way. When you smell it, it has a certain aroma; when you bite into it and chew then swallow, it has a certain texture. In other words, it's a multi-sensory experience.

Sadly, a lot of people with weight problems or diet issues don't look at it that way. They see it really just as some sort of pitstop to load up on calories, and then they move on to the next pitstop, and on and on it goes.

You have to change your mindset regarding your food. Make each meal a celebration. This means truly enjoying your food.

How do you do this? Well, the first step is nothing more basic than simply deciding to chew your food more. Seriously. Make a conscious effort to chew your food a certain number of times.

After you get used to that, just allow yourself to chew food for a longer period of time. What do you think will happen? Well, if you're like most people, this would lead to smaller portions because you actually taste and enjoy your food better. This means that you don't need more of it to get the same sense of appreciation.

Truly savoring your food means giving it enough time. You don't rush through it. You make it a ritual that takes a long time to unwind and truly savor. As a result, you require smaller portions.

Finally, try to eat with friends and family. When you enjoy a meal with friends and family members, you redirect your attention from simply filling your belly to satiety.

How come? Well, your first priority is to talk, socialize, and enjoy each other's company. It's not to gorge yourself so your body gets used to this new definition of satiety.

Again, this is just a component of a larger picture. The larger picture here is that you have to look at each meal as a celebration that you truly enjoy with all your senses.

Get Out from Under Emotional Eating

A key part of adopting a fat-burning lifestyle is to identify comfort eating patterns.

I don't care how slim you are or how problematic or how easy weight loss is to you. All of us suffer from some level of comfort eating or another. All of us. I can make that claim with a straight face.

Because the reason why a lot of people have issues with eating is because they have some sort of **emotional association with eating** that's not all that healthy. And a lot of this eventually leads back to some sort of comfort eating pattern.

You eat not because you need to. You eat because you associate it with the release of serotonin in your brain that makes you deal with life much better.

For example, a lot of people eat because they're stressed. A lot of people eat comfort foods because they feel down or challenged. They feel anxious or uncertain.

Do you see the problem here? You're loading up on calories precisely at the point in time where you should avoid calories and deal with your problem head on.

Your problem is emotional, not physiological. But the problem is, people associate that nice burst of serotonin when they eat with the "solution" to their stress and emotional roller coaster.

To get out from under this pattern which can easily become addictive, you must identify your comfort eating patterns. When do you normally eat for comfort? What needs to happen for you to engage in this type of eating behavior? In other words, what are your "triggers" that make you turn to food for comfort?

Second, look at the stress patterns that you go through and your eating choices. Once you see these patterns, you will then be able to better prepare to deal with them.

When you experience them, disrupt these by eating less calorie-dense foods. You're still eating, but the amount of calories that you are ingesting into your system does less damage. What you are doing is finding less calorie-dense foods to replace your comfort foods.

Similarly, you could disrupt by choosing to cope by doing something else.

If you're feeling stressed, you don't necessarily have to raid the fridge and gorge on a thick slice of German chocolate cake. You can do deep, slow breathing. You can simply choose to count slowly. You can drink water.

Another alternative is to simply just get up and walk. You'd be surprised as to how effective these changes can be in disrupting what would otherwise seem to be like an iron clad habit.

Be Aware of and Take Control of Your Snacking

A lot of people can do much of the things that I've described above, but unfortunately, a lot of them would find the following quite challenging.

It's one thing to be on the lookout for main meals because these are the main "dietary" events of your day, but unless you become aware of your snacking habits, you're not going to make much progress. Why? You might end up shifting a lot of your calorie intake to your snacks.

So how do you take control of your snacking patterns? Well, first of all, you should decide to savor your snacks.

I'm not saying you should cut out snacks or stop eating snacks. You can do what you're doing before, but take the time while you are eating your snack to truly savor it.

Instead of just running through that package of potato chips, savor each chip. Taste the fat. Taste the salt. Enjoy the texture.

When you do this, you control your eating process. You smell it, you touch it, you taste it. It's like you're eating several times with one bite.

Because normally, when people eat, they just look for the taste. They experience the food once, in one dimension and as fast as they can.

When you make a conscious effort to smell, touch, taste, and really experience the snack item, you control the process. And this leads you to reframing your snacking into an experience.

Instead of something that you just **must** do, it becomes something that you **choose** to do. Because let's face it, if you think that something is an activity that you must do, it's more likely that you will race through it. And when you race through it, you have absolutely no portion control. You simply eat until the package is empty.

But when you shift your mindset and you think that this is something that you choose to do, you start looking at it as an experience. You start looking at it as an option that you can sit down, enjoy, and relish. And portion control becomes much easier.

Chapter 5 – Burn Fat by Increasing Your Daily Practical Activity Levels

This chapter is going to involve a topic that a lot of people on diets find rather uncomfortable. I am of course talking about physical activity.

The general idea most people have is that if they want to burn fat, they necessarily have to sign up for a gym membership and put in the time hitting the weights, pumping iron, and sweating buckets.

As you can well imagine, a lot of people look at that picture as something involving pain, sacrifice and, let's face it, some sort of torture or another.

I really can't blame people because that is an alien experience. That's not how you normally experience your life. That's not your normal activity level. But people think that if you're serious about burning fat and losing weight, they must go crazy and hit the gym.

Well, let me tell you, when people adopt that drastic and abrupt lifestyle change, that change isn't usually permanent. They end up going back to their previous physical activity level, and guess what? That's right - the fat comes back.

If you're sick and tired of losing weight by exercising and then getting it back as your lifestyle changes, this is the chapter for you.

Quick Recap: How Your Body Burns Fat

Your body burns fat when you increase your body's physical activity. That's the bottom line. Why? Increased physical activity requires more calories.

Your body needs calories for its energy requirements. When this happens, your body will first tap the amount of sugar in your bloodstream. Once that's gone, it will raid the amount of sugar in your liver. Once that's tapped, your body then goes through a transition called Ketosis.

Assuming that you don't eat any sugar in the form of carbohydrates after your blood sugar levels are depleted, your body will start to tap your fat cells for energy. This happens in a low carb setting where you ingest less than 50 grams of carbohydrates per day.

Now, don't get too excited. This doesn't happen overnight. For you to make that ketosis switch, you must stick with it for the long term.

But the good news is, once you are more ketogenic than otherwise, your body is now primed to burn that nasty layer of fat all around your body, especially that spare tire you have in your midsection, for energy.

Adopt Gradual Long-Term Fat Burning Daily Activities

As awesome as ketosis is, a lot of people think that they should just jumpstart. They should just jump in with both feet, hit the gym, or run five miles every day, and ketosis will take care of the rest.

I'm happy to report that they're absolutely correct. If you increase your physical activities and you cut down on sugar or you cut down on calories, you will lose weight quickly.

The problem is, as I've repeatedly said in this book, is not weight loss. Weight loss will happen. The problem is sustainability. Can you keep the fat off?

And I'm sad to report that if you just get all pumped up one day and just hit the gym and start running and doing extensive cardio exercises on a daily basis, you will lose weight. The problem is, you're not really setting in motion any long-term changes that will ensure that the weight stays off.

It is no surprise that a lot of people who go on shows like The Biggest Loser end up getting fatter. I know that sounds crazy because a lot of those people looked really good at the end of the show.

They start out with 200 extra pounds, and then they slimmed down. They looked really good. And then when you visit them 6 months or maybe a year later, they weigh even more than when they began the show.

The real solution is less sexy. The real solution involves adopting gradual long-term fat burning daily activities.

There's nothing sexy about this because it's all about increasing physical activity that has nothing to do with the gym. It is not in-your-face, it is not blatant, it is not flamboyant or flagrant. Instead, it involves day to day small changes in your physical activity levels that add up to a lot.

What are we talking about? It's all about simply increasing your physical activity on a day to day basis, like lifting more bags instead of buying something that shifts the weight of the bag.

For example, you can buy specialized luggage with wheels that would shift a lot of the weight of the stuff you're lifting. What if you just choose to lift grocery bags or your luggage for your office the natural way?

It might seem a little bit inconvenient, but it's a minor inconvenience. Eventually, you get used to it. But let me tell you, that small change in your daily lifting activities can burn more calories.

Similarly, you can park far away from the entrance of your office. It may seem small, but each and every footstep you add to your daily routine leads to more calories burned.

You probably already heard of taking the stairs instead of the elevator. Now, the good news is that you don't have to be a hero about this. You can just choose to take one set of stairs. You don't have to start with ten. This is not some sort of ironman event.

You can start low and slow. Just take the stairs for one flight. Once you get used to it, increase it to two flights. Then three.

Similarly, you can choose to stand up from your work cubicle and walk around the office. Now, you may be thinking to yourself, "Wouldn't people notice? Wouldn't it look like I'm just wasting my time or I'm goofing off at work?"

Well, you must understand that in any typical American office, there are usually hard copies of papers that are shifted or shuffled off from one department to another. In fact, depending on the nature of your job, you're probably shuffling off a lot of these pieces paper and having the office messenger do it.

Well, you can boost the amount of physical activity in your day to day routine by simply taking these papers to other departments yourself. That's right.

Instead of having other staff members do it, do it yourself. It's nice, it's quick, people are not going to notice, but you end up burning more calories.
Need to send a colleague a message? Write it up, print it out and hand-deliver it instead of sending it electronically.

If you take public transportation to and from work, get off either one stop before or one stop after your normal closest stop to your office and walk the rest of the way in.

And the best part to all of this is that if you choose to do these things on a day to day basis, you eventually get used to it. So, your overall calorie burn rate goes up tremendously and it doesn't look and feel like you're punishing yourself or doing something out of the ordinary.

Similarly, talking to people while you're walking increases the amount of distance you cover. Because when you're talking to people while you're walking around the office or on a trail, you don't put any attention to the fact that you're walking. It doesn't seem like a chore. It doesn't seem like such a deviation from your normal routine.

Finally, it's a good idea to adopt a morning physical activity routine. Again, don't freak out. I'm not saying that you should just jog around the block for ten miles. By simply just walking around or walking your dog first thing in the morning, you can do yourself a very big favor.

If you want a little more calorie burn, carry some weight while you are walking. It could be a weighted vest, belt, ankle and/or wrist weights – whatever. And swing your arms while walking. That burns even more calories. Once you get used to that amount of weight, increase it by a pound or two at a time.

The truth is, low and slow will do it. Let me repeat that. Low and slow will do it.

Easy Does It

Boosting your physical activity levels doesn't have to be dramatic. You're not trying to impress anybody.

What will truly impress people is not you losing weight as if overnight, and then gaining it all back. That doesn't impress people. Do you know what will impress people? Losing weight and then keeping it off - sustainability.

And the best thing about doing things low and slow is that you put yourself on the road to doing exactly that. You're focusing on sustainability. You're not shooting for that shock and awe "one-time big time" kind of effect.

Instead of obsessing about how many miles you walk or how long you work out or how much weight you lift, you should shift your main metric for physical activity. Your main metric should be on how quickly your new routine sticks or how "deeply ingrained" it becomes.

Conclusion

I know a lot of the topics that I raised here seem easier said than done. Well, let me tell you, there are a lot of big changes that all of us must make that are easier said than done.

The problem is, these ideas, no matter how well developed and effective they may be for other people, are not going to change our lives until we choose to do something.

What is that? We need to choose to do it. It really is that basic.

Everything that I've shared with you in this book is not going to change your life or do you any good unless you *choose* to do it.

Pay close attention to that directive. Choose. This is a choice. You have chosen to ***not do*** it in the past. Now is your opportunity to choose to ***do*** it – now.

You can choose to stick with the results that you're getting now. But I'm sure the fact that you're reading this book, indicates that you're not very happy with the results that you're getting.

Maybe you're feeling desperate. Maybe you feel that no matter how hard to try, nothing seems to change. Maybe you're anxious. Maybe you're feeling lost.

Well, now is the time to do something about it. But the key is to choose to do it. In other words, you need to take action.

I've got some bad news for you. Taking action doesn't mean mentally realizing that you have to do something. Hey, anybody can do that.

Choosing to do something means you have to decide on a date. This must be a date or a start time that you cannot simply postpone.

You're not doing something or deciding something when you choose a date that you can conveniently disregard. Decide on a date that you know you can stick to. This is not as easy as you would think.

A lot of people choose a date that is so close to the present that they end up freaking themselves out. It's so close that they're so intimidated, so they end up postponing it.

Healthy Lifestyle Newsletter

Similarly, other people choose a date that is so far into the future that they end up filling in that time. So, by the time the start date rolls around, they're just as unprepared as the day they set the date.

Don't play any of these games on yourself. Decide on a date that you know you can start on. When that date comes, do one thing and one thing alone: start.

The good thing about all of this is that you don't have to start like a Kentucky Derby thoroughbred. You don't have to get out of the gate like a lightning bolt. You can just start one step at a time, one choice at a time, one meal at a time.

Let's put it this way, if you make one 6-inch step forward, you're still half a foot better off than when you began.

Choose to start. When you've started, that's when the opposition begins. Your mind and your body will try to play tricks on you.

Remember, you're trying to regress to a mean. You're trying to go back to what you're accustomed to, so choose to be aware of these tricks.

I've already exposed them in the previous chapters of this book. Go ahead and review them and decide not to play these tricks on yourself.

Finally, as you move forward, allow yourself to feel good about any progress you make. A lot of people sabotage themselves because they expect amazing results the moment they start.

Well, this is not your typical diet book. This is not the Atkins diet where you can see 5, 10, or even 15-pounds of weight loss in as little as a week. Don't set yourself up for failure. You're much more precious than that. You did not gain the weight you want to lose overnight nor should you expect to lose it overnight. It will take work, time, and a positive can-do mental mindset. You body will do what the mind tells it to do ... you just have to tell it to do the right thing. Weight loss is as much or even more a mental struggle as it is physical.

Allow yourself to feel good about any progress you make. If you used to eat large portions and now you're eating smaller portions, feel good about that. If you used to snack throughout the day and now you can tell that you're snacking more purposely and less often, feel good about that.

It's all about choice. And choose to be aware. And when you become aware, allow yourself to feel good about it.

By following all these tips, you will be able to adopt a lifestyle that burns fat instead of desperately jumping from one diet to another. In other words, you totally change your weight loss orientation so that the weight loss becomes sustainable.

I wish you nothing but the greatest success.

For More Information …

For more information on the topics of the words highlighted in this book, copy the link and past it into Amazon.com:

- Ketogenic Diet - https://www.amazon.com/gp/product/169538427X

- Paleo diet - https://www.amazon.com/gp/product/1534601708

- Lifestyle - https://www.amazon.com/gp/product/1546424660

- Mindset - https://www.amazon.com/gp/product/1070768383

- Emotional association with eating -

  https://www.amazon.com/gp/product/1512064971

About the Author

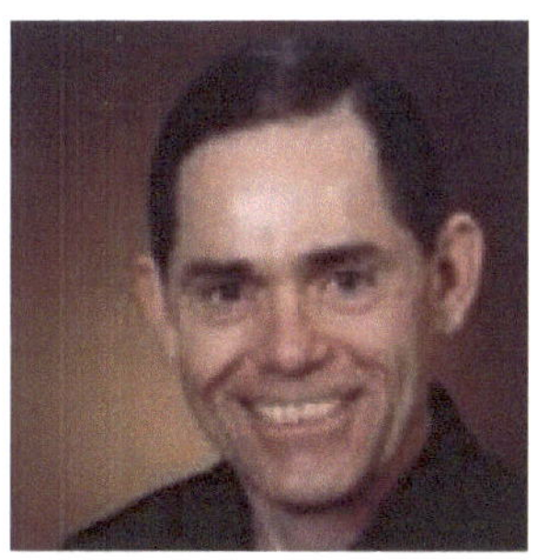

I have published numerous books on Amazon (both for Kindle and in paperback), along with other publishing platforms.

While most of my books are on health and fitness in general, I also write on baby boomer and older citizen health issues and have a recent interest in creating and printing journals/ planners and other printable products.

Besides my own writing, I also ghostwrite ebooks, books, reports, articles, blogs and do Kindle conversions for clients on a variety of topics.

Go to my website at http://ronknesswriting.com for more information or to submit a quote. For a complete list of my books, go to https://www.amazon.com/Ron-Kness/e/B0072M6PYO.

Today my wife and I are retired from our careers and live in Queen Creek, AZ. I now write as a retirement business where you'll find me happily sitting in my office typing away on my laptop as I work on my next book or ghostwriting project . . . that is if we are not traveling on a cruise ship - our new-found mode of travel.